Benign Prostatic Hypertrophy

A Beginner's 3-Step Plan for Managing BPH with and Nutrition, with Sample Recipes and a Meal Plan

copyright © 2022 Larry Jamesonn

All rights reserved No part of this book may be reproduced, or stored in a retrieval system, or transmitted in any form or by any means, electronic, mechanical, photocopying, recording, or otherwise, without express written permission of the publisher.

Disclaimer

By reading this disclaimer, you are accepting the terms of the disclaimer in full. If you disagree with this disclaimer, please do not read the guide.

All of the content within this guide is provided for informational and educational purposes only, and should not be accepted as independent medical or other professional advice. The author is not a doctor, physician, nurse, mental health provider, or registered nutritionist/dietician. Therefore, using and reading this guide does not establish any form of a physician-patient relationship.

Always consult with a physician or another qualified health provider with any issues or questions you might have regarding any sort of medical condition. Do not ever disregard any qualified professional medical advice or delay seeking that advice because of anything you have read in this guide. The information in this guide is not intended to be any sort of medical advice and should not be used in lieu of any medical advice by a licensed and qualified medical professional.

The information in this guide has been compiled from a variety of known sources. However, the author cannot attest to or guarantee the accuracy of each source and thus should not be held liable for any errors or omissions.

You acknowledge that the publisher of this guide will not be held liable for any loss or damage of any kind incurred as a result of this guide or the reliance on any information provided within this guide. You acknowledge and agree that you assume all risk and responsibility for any action you undertake in response to the information in this guide.

Using this guide does not guarantee any particular result (e.g., weight loss or a cure). By reading this guide, you acknowledge that there are no guarantees to any specific outcome or results you can expect.

All product names, diet plans, or names used in this guide are for identification purposes only and are the property of their respective owners. The use of these names does not imply endorsement. All other trademarks cited herein are the property of their respective owners.

Where applicable, this guide is not intended to be a substitute for the original work of this diet plan and is, at most, a supplement to the original work for this diet plan and never a direct substitute. This guide is a personal expression of the facts of that diet plan.

Where applicable, persons shown in the cover images are stock photography models and the publisher has obtained the rights to use the images through license agreements with third-party stock image companies.

Table of Contents

Introduction   7
Benign Prostatic Hypertrophy   10
    What causes benign prostatic hypertrophy?   11
    What are some common symptoms?   12
Diagnosing BPH   15
Treatment and Prevention   17
    Prevention of BPH   18
    Are there any alternative treatments for BPH?   19
    Lifestyle Changes to Manage the BPH   21
Managing BPH Through Diet   24
    Principles of a BPH-Friendly Diet   24
    Benefits of BPH- Friendly Diet   26
    Potential Disadvantages   28
A 3-Step Plan to Manage BPH Through Diet   30
    Step 1: Gradual Elimination of BPH-Unfriendly Foods   30
    Step 2: Opt for Healthier Substitutes and Reduce Consumption Where Necessary   33
    Step 3: Enrich Your Diet Through Creativity and Planning   36
Foods to Eat and to Avoid   40
    Foods to Eat   40
    Foods to Avoid   41
Sample 7-Day Meal Plan   43
    Tips for Meal Planning and Food Preparation   46
Sample Recipes   49
    Chicken Rotisserie and Vegetable Broth   50
    Ikarian Stew with Black-Eyed Peas   51
    Lentil Stew   53
    Vegetable Broth   55
    Broccoli Soup   57

Chicken Soup	58
Salmon Soup	59
Salmon and Asparagus	60
Seafood Stew	61
Salmon with Avocados and Brussels Sprouts	62
Baked Salmon	65
Zucchini and Celery Greens Soup	67
Chia Seed and Strawberry Pudding	69
Fruity Berry Spinach Smoothie	70
Roasted Broccoli and Salmon	71
Tomato and Spinach Quinoa Salad	73
Lemon-Garlic Baked Salmon	75
Chicken and Broccoli Stir-Fry	76
Avocado and Bean Wrap	78
Conclusion	**80**
FAQ	**84**
References and Helpful Links	**87**

Introduction

Dealing with Benign Prostatic Hyperplasia (BPH) can seem overwhelming. For those afflicted by its uncomfortable symptoms, finding effective ways to manage the condition becomes crucial. Diet plays a key role among the various strategies, significantly affecting the severity of BPH's impact. This guide is designed to show how wise dietary decisions can markedly improve life quality for people struggling with BPH.

The link between our diet and health is well-documented, yet the specifics of how food choices affect BPH symptoms might not be widely known. Certain foods and nutrients hold power over prostate health, influencing everything from irritation levels to symptom severity. Recognizing the potential of a carefully considered diet offers hope and a new avenue for symptom management.

Gaining insights into which foods might benefit or exacerbate BPH symptoms is invaluable. This guide breaks down the essentials, from the antioxidant-rich fruits and vegetables that support your health, to the potential pitfalls of consuming too much red meat and dairy. Beyond just what to eat, it covers hydration's role, the importance of healthy fats, and considerations for supplements. The aim is to equip you with knowledge, simplifying dietary decisions in the context of BPH.

Envisioning a day with fewer BPH symptoms because of dietary changes brings a sense of hope. It's not about restrictive diets but finding a harmonious balance that nurtures prostate health while still delighting in what you eat. The universal longing for symptom relief among BPH sufferers can be addressed through thoughtful dietary choices, making better health an achievable goal.

In this guide, we will talk about the following;

- Benign Prostatic Hypertrophy
- Causes, Symptoms, and Diagnosis of Benign Prostatic Hypertrophy
- Treatment and Preventions
- Lifestyle Changes to Manage BPH
- Managing BPH through Diet
- Principles and Benefits of the BPH-Friendly Diet
- A 3-Step Plan to Manage BPH Through Diet
- Foods to Eat and To Avoid
- 7-Day Sample Meal Plan and Recipes

We encourage you to continue reading, explore the dietary modifications suggested, and consider how these changes can be woven into your everyday life for enhanced prostate health.

The relationship between diet and health has never been more relevant, especially for those managing Benign Prostatic Hyperplasia. By focusing on dietary modifications, this guide provides a ray of hope and practical steps for individuals looking to mitigate their symptoms through better food choices.

Benign Prostatic Hypertrophy

Benign prostatic hyperplasia or hypertrophy (BPH) is the common term for an enlargement of the prostate gland in men. The prostate gland is approximately the size of a walnut and is located in front of the rectum and underneath the urinary bladder.

The function of this gland is to add fluids to the seminal fluid during ejaculation. With BPH, the prostate enlarges and puts pressure on the urethra, which can make it difficult to urinate. This can lead to frequent nighttime urination and may cause a weak or interrupted urine stream.

As a man ages, some of his prostate cells may develop mutations (abnormalities) and begin to multiply rapidly. A group of these abnormal cells forms a distinct area within the otherwise normal gland called an adenoma or benign prostatic hyperplasia, which can continue to expand and compress surrounding structures such as the urethra (urinary tube).

The compressive effect on the urethra is what causes most symptoms associated with BPH such as increased urination frequency, urgency, intermittency, incomplete voiding, straining at the end of urination, weak urinary stream, etc.

Enlargement can cause urinary symptoms including frequent urination, the urgency to urinate, weak or interrupted flow, and pain with urination. Prostate enlargement can cause sexual problems including erectile dysfunction.

What causes benign prostatic hypertrophy?

Benign prostatic hypertrophy (BPH), also known as prostate gland enlargement, is a common condition as men get older. It's mainly caused by changes in hormone balance and cell growth. Here are some of the key factors involved:

1. *Aging*: The risk of BPH increases with age, particularly after the age of 50. It's believed that aging-related hormonal changes may contribute to the enlargement of the prostate.
2. *Hormonal Changes*: With age, the balance of hormones in the body changes. An increase in estrogen (relative to testosterone) levels has been associated with BPH. The prostate gland partly depends on testosterone to function normally, and alterations in these hormone levels can lead to prostate growth.
3. *Cellular Growth Factors*: Changes in cell growth factors and other cell signaling pathways can also contribute to the proliferation of prostate cells, leading to an enlarged prostate.

4. ***Genetic Factors***: There's evidence that genetics may play a role in the development of BPH. Men with a family history of prostate problems are more likely to develop BPH.
5. ***Lifestyle Factors***: While less directly implicated, factors such as diet, exercise, and overall health may influence the risk or severity of BPH.

The exact mechanism by which these factors contribute to BPH is complex and involves multiple pathways. Essentially, it's a combination of aging, hormonal changes, genetic predispositions, and possibly lifestyle factors that lead to the benign enlargement of the prostate gland.

What are some common symptoms?

Benign prostatic hypertrophy (BPH) can lead to a range of urinary symptoms due to the enlarged prostate pressing on the urethra and affecting bladder control. Some of the common symptoms include:

1. ***Frequent Urination***: This involves the need to urinate more often than is typical for the individual, particularly noticeable during nighttime hours (nocturia), which may disrupt sleep and affect daily life.
2. ***The Urgency to Urinate***: Individuals may experience a sudden, overwhelming urge to urinate, which can be

both inconvenient and embarrassing, especially if access to a restroom is not immediate.
3. **_Difficulty Starting Urination_**: Some people find it challenging to initiate urination. This issue often involves straining to start the flow of urine, indicating a possible obstruction in the urinary tract or an issue with bladder muscles.
4. **_Weak Urine Stream_**: The flow of urine may be noticeably weaker or intermittent, with the stream stopping and starting unpredictably. This can lead to prolonged times spent in the restroom and a feeling of frustration.
5. **_Dribbling at the End of Urination_**: After the main flow of urine has stopped, small amounts may continue to dribble out. This can be uncomfortable and may require extra hygiene measures to manage.
6. **_Incomplete Emptying_**: There can be a persistent sensation that the bladder is not fully emptied, despite having just urinated. This feeling can be both uncomfortable and anxiety-inducing, as it feels like one needs to urinate again soon after leaving the restroom.
7. **_Urinary Retention_**: This is characterized by a significant difficulty in urinating despite the urge, which can lead to serious discomfort, bladder infections, and in severe cases, require medical intervention to relieve the retention.

8. ***Urinary Tract Infections (UTIs)***: Due to the challenges associated with fully emptying the bladder, individuals may face an increased risk of developing urinary tract infections. UTIs can cause additional symptoms such as pain, burning during urination, and fever, further complicating the condition.

While these symptoms are common with BPH, they can also indicate other conditions. It's important for individuals experiencing these symptoms to consult a healthcare provider for an accurate diagnosis and appropriate treatment.

Diagnosing BPH

To diagnose Benign Prostatic Hyperplasia (BPH), doctors will first rule out other potential causes of urinary symptoms, such as infections or prostate cancer. The diagnostic process typically involves several steps:

- *Medical History Assessment*: This includes questions about urinary habits (frequency, dribbling post-urination, pain during urination or ejaculation), sexual health, and any medications, herbs, or supplements being taken.
- *Physical Examination*: A Digital Rectal Exam (DRE) is performed to manually check the prostate gland for size, shape, and texture. Additionally, a Transrectal Ultrasound (TRUS) may be used to obtain detailed images of the prostate and assess bladder outlet obstruction by measuring the resistance at the bladder outlet.
- *Diagnostic Tests*: Blood tests are conducted to identify signs of inflammation, infection, or anemia. A 24-hour urine collection test helps check for blood, creatinine levels (indicating kidney function), electrolyte balance,

and prostate-specific antigen levels, which increase in response to prostate inflammation.

- ***Further Evaluation with TRUS***: If BPH symptoms persist without evidence of a urinary tract infection, a TRUS might be requested. This procedure is not only helpful in evaluating BPH but also plays a role in staging bladder tumors, guiding biopsies, and assisting in the identification of tumor types during surgery.

Through these comprehensive steps, doctors can accurately diagnose BPH and differentiate it from other conditions with similar symptoms.

Treatment and Prevention

Treatment options for BPH vary depending on the severity of symptoms, ranging from lifestyle adjustments and medications to surgical interventions:

1. ***Lifestyle Changes***: For mild symptoms, changes such as reducing fluid intake before bed, limiting caffeine and alcohol, practicing double voiding (urinating, then urinating again a few minutes later) to empty the bladder, and doing pelvic floor exercises can help manage symptoms.
2. ***Medications***:
    - Alpha-blockers (e.g., tamsulosin, alfuzosin) relax the muscles of the bladder neck, and prostate, improving urine flow.
    - 5-alpha reductase inhibitors (e.g., finasteride, dutasteride) reduce prostate size by blocking hormonal changes that cause prostate growth.
    - Phosphodiesterase-5 inhibitors (e.g., tadalafil) used for erectile dysfunction can also alleviate BPH symptoms.

3. **Minimally Invasive Procedures**: When medication is ineffective, procedures like transurethral resection of the prostate (TURP), laser therapy, or prostatic urethral lift can be considered to remove or reduce prostate tissue and relieve urinary symptoms.
4. **Surgery**: In severe cases, where there's significant bladder damage, recurrent blood in the urine, or kidney problems, surgery might be recommended to remove prostate tissue.

Prevention of BPH

While it's not always possible to prevent BPH due to its strong link with aging and genetic factors, certain lifestyle practices can help lower the risk or mitigate the severity of symptoms:

1. **Regular Exercise**: Maintaining an active lifestyle can help reduce the risk of developing BPH and alleviate symptoms.
2. **Healthy Diet**: Eating a balanced diet rich in fruits, vegetables, and whole grains can support overall health, including prostate health.
3. **Maintain a Healthy Weight**: Obesity is associated with an increased risk of BPH; thus, maintaining a healthy weight can help prevent or reduce symptoms.

4. ***Limit Fluid Intake Before Bed***: Reducing fluid consumption in the evening can help decrease nighttime urination.
5. ***Avoid or Limit Caffeine and Alcohol***: These can exacerbate symptoms by increasing urine production or making it more difficult to empty the bladder.
6. ***Regular Check-ups***: Regular visits to the doctor for prostate screenings can help detect problems early, making them easier to manage.

By combining preventative measures with appropriate treatment strategies, individuals can effectively manage BPH symptoms and maintain a good quality of life.

Are there any alternative treatments for BPH?

There are several alternative treatments for Benign Prostatic Hyperplasia (BPH) that many individuals explore alongside or instead of conventional medical treatments. These alternatives focus on natural supplements, lifestyle modifications, and other non-surgical methods:

1. ***Saw Palmetto***: One of the most popular herbal supplements for BPH, Saw Palmetto is believed to help reduce urinary symptoms associated with an enlarged prostate. However, its effectiveness varies, and more research is needed to conclusively determine its benefits.

2. ***Beta-Sitosterol***: This plant-based substance found in fruits, vegetables, nuts, and seeds has shown some promise in improving urinary flow rate and reducing the amount of urine left in the bladder after urination.
3. ***Pygeum***: Derived from the bark of the African plum tree, pygeum has been used to treat various urinary issues. It's thought to help reduce BPH symptoms, although evidence is mixed and more research is needed.
4. ***Rye Grass Pollen Extract***: Some studies suggest that rye grass pollen extract can improve symptoms of BPH, such as nighttime urination and incomplete emptying of the bladder.
5. ***Stinging Nettle***: Often used in combination with other herbs like saw palmetto, stinging nettle may help relieve symptoms of BPH, though more high-quality studies are needed.
6. ***Zinc Supplements***: Zinc plays a role in prostate health, and some research indicates that zinc supplementation might be beneficial for BPH, though the findings are not conclusive.
7. ***Lifestyle Changes***: Regular exercise, maintaining a healthy weight, reducing stress, and practicing bladder training techniques can also support overall prostate health and mitigate BPH symptoms.
8. ***Mindfulness and Stress Reduction***: Techniques like mindfulness-based stress reduction (MBSR) and yoga

may help improve quality of life and reduce BPH symptoms by managing stress levels, which can influence symptoms.
9. *Acupuncture*: Some men find relief from BPH symptoms through acupuncture, a traditional Chinese medicine technique that involves inserting thin needles into specific points on the body.

It's important to note that while these alternative treatments can offer relief for some individuals, they may not work for everyone and can interact with conventional medications. Therefore, it's crucial to consult with a healthcare provider before starting any alternative treatments for BPH to ensure they are safe and suitable for your specific health situation.

Lifestyle Changes to Manage the BPH

Managing Benign Prostatic Hyperplasia (BPH) effectively often involves making several lifestyle changes aimed at alleviating symptoms and improving quality of life. Here are some recommended changes:

1. **Adjust Your Diet**
- Reduce caffeine and alcohol intake: These can irritate the bladder and increase symptoms.
- Drink plenty of water: Stay hydrated but try to limit fluid intake in the evening to reduce nighttime urination.

- Focus on a balanced diet: Incorporate fruits, vegetables, whole grains, and lean proteins to support overall health.

2. **Manage Fluid Intake**
- Limit fluids before bedtime: To minimize nocturia (frequent night-time urination), avoid drinking fluids 2-3 hours before bedtime.
- Spread out fluid intake: Drink fluids throughout the day in moderate amounts instead of large quantities at once.

3. **Exercise Regularly**
- Maintain a healthy weight: Extra weight can put additional pressure on the bladder.
- Physical activity: Regular exercise can help manage symptoms. However, avoid activities that put extra pressure on the prostate, like bike riding.

4. **Pelvic Floor Exercises**

   Kegel exercises: Strengthening the pelvic floor muscles can help manage incontinence related to BPH.

5. **Urinary Habits**
- Double voiding: After urinating, wait a few moments and then try to go again to ensure the bladder is empty.
- Schedule bathroom visits: Go to the bathroom at regular times to train the bladder.

6. **Avoid Certain Medications**

   Some over-the-counter medications for colds or allergies can exacerbate BPH symptoms. It's important to consult with a healthcare provider about the safety of any medications.

7. **Stay Warm**

   Cold weather can sometimes worsen BPH symptoms, so keeping warm may help.

8. **Stress Management**

   Stress can aggravate symptoms of BPH. Techniques such as meditation, yoga, or other relaxation practices can be beneficial.

Implementing these lifestyle changes can significantly help manage BPH symptoms. However, it's always important to work closely with a healthcare provider to monitor the condition and adjust treatments as necessary.

In the next chapter, we'll discuss what to eat for prostate health.

Managing BPH Through Diet

Managing your diet is an important aspect of supporting overall prostate health and managing the symptoms of BPH. While there is no specific BPH diet, making certain dietary changes can help reduce inflammation in the body and potentially alleviate symptoms.

Principles of a BPH-Friendly Diet

Here are some Principles of a BPH-friendly diet to consider:

- *Eat plenty of fruits and vegetables*: Consuming a variety of fruits and vegetables enriches your diet with essential antioxidants, vitamins, and minerals. These nutrients are crucial for combating inflammation throughout the body, supporting overall health and well-being.
- *Incorporate plant-based proteins*: Including plant-based sources of protein such as beans, lentils, nuts, and seeds in your diet not only provides you with vital nutrients but also serves as a healthier alternative to animal-based proteins. Animal proteins can

sometimes lead to increased inflammation, so opting for plant-based options can be beneficial.
- ***Limit or avoid alcohol and caffeine***: Both alcohol and caffeine have the potential to irritate the bladder, which can exacerbate the symptoms of Benign Prostatic Hyperplasia (BPH). By reducing or completely avoiding these substances, individuals may notice a significant alleviation in discomfort and improvement in symptoms.
- ***Choose healthy fats***: Incorporating foods high in Omega-3 fatty acids, such as fish, avocados, and nuts, into your diet can have a positive impact on your health. Omega-3s are well-known for their anti-inflammatory properties, which can be particularly beneficial for maintaining prostate health and reducing inflammation.
- ***Reduce red meat and dairy intake***: Consumption of red meat and dairy products has been linked to increased inflammation in the body, which may aggravate symptoms associated with BPH. It is advisable to limit or avoid these foods and explore alternative dietary options to help manage symptoms more effectively.
- ***Stay hydrated***: Maintaining adequate hydration is key to minimizing bladder irritation and promoting a healthy urine flow. Drinking sufficient water throughout the day helps flush toxins from the bladder

and reduces the risk of urinary tract infections, which can worsen BPH symptoms.

Overall, a diet that is rich in whole, unprocessed foods and low in inflammatory substances can help promote prostate health and manage BPH symptoms.

Benefits of BPH- Friendly Diet

Following a BPH-friendly diet can have numerous benefits, including:

- *Improved Urinary Symptoms*: Adopting a diet low in inflammatory foods while being rich in essential nutrients can significantly alleviate the uncomfortable symptoms associated with Benign Prostatic Hyperplasia (BPH), including urinary frequency, urgency, and nocturia. This dietary approach focuses on reducing inflammation and supporting the urinary tract's overall health.
- *Overall Health Enhancement*: Beyond targeting BPH symptoms, this nutritious diet champions general wellness by aiding in weight management, bolstering heart health, and diminishing the risk of developing chronic conditions such as diabetes and hypertension. It's a holistic approach to health that benefits every aspect of the individual's well-being.
- *Increased Energy Levels*: By ensuring a balanced intake of vitamins, minerals, and other vital nutrients,

this diet aims to provide a more consistent and sustained energy supply throughout the day. This boost in energy levels significantly enhances overall well-being and lifestyle quality, allowing individuals to engage more actively in their daily activities without the usual mid-day slumps.

- ***Better Digestive Health***: A high intake of dietary fiber from a variety of fruits, vegetables, and whole grains is a cornerstone of this diet, promoting robust digestive health. This is particularly beneficial for individuals with BPH since a well-functioning digestive system can help prevent constipation, a condition known to exacerbate BPH symptoms. A healthy digestive system also aids in the absorption of nutrients, contributing to overall health.
- ***Long-Term Prostate Health***: By embracing healthy eating habits, individuals can contribute significantly to their long-term prostate health. A diet rich in antioxidants, omega-3 fatty acids, and phytonutrients supports the prostate's health and may help slow the progression of conditions such as BPH. This preventive approach emphasizes the importance of diet in maintaining prostate health and potentially reducing the need for medical interventions in the future.

By making small changes to your diet and incorporating more BPH-friendly foods, you can improve your prostate health and overall well-being. It is always important to consult with a healthcare professional before making any significant changes to your diet or lifestyle. They can provide personalized recommendations and guidance for managing BPH symptoms.

Potential Disadvantages

Adopting a BPH-friendly diet, which is often rich in fruits, vegetables, lean proteins, and whole grains while low in red meats and high-fat dairy products, comes with numerous benefits for managing symptoms of Benign Prostatic Hyperplasia (BPH). However, like any dietary adjustment, there are potential disadvantages to consider, though these are generally outweighed by the benefits:

- *Initial Adjustment Period*: Switching to a BPH-friendly diet may require a period of adjustment, especially for individuals accustomed to diets high in processed foods or red meat. This transition can be challenging and might involve a learning curve.
- *Potential Dietary Restrictions*: For some, a BPH-friendly diet might mean cutting back on certain favorite foods or beverages that are known to exacerbate BPH symptoms, such as caffeine, spicy foods, and alcohol. This could feel restrictive.
- *Increased Meal Planning and Preparation*: Incorporating a wider variety of fruits, vegetables, and whole grains often means spending more time

planning meals and preparing food, which could be a significant change for those used to more convenient eating options.

- ***Cost Considerations***: Depending on one's location and access to fresh produce, adopting a diet rich in fruits and vegetables can lead to increased grocery bills, especially if opting for organic or specialty food items.

While these potential disadvantages may seem daunting, it's important to remember the long-term benefits of a BPH-friendly diet in managing symptoms and promoting overall health. Additionally, with some adjustments and planning, these potential downsides can be minimized or overcome entirely.

A 3-Step Plan to Manage BPH Through Diet

Adjusting to a new diet following a diagnosis of Benign Prostatic Hyperplasia (BPH) can be challenging. This three-step plan is designed to simplify the transition, allowing you and your family to gradually adapt without feeling overwhelmed. It's advisable to spread this adjustment over two to three weeks to ease into the new dietary lifestyle comfortably.

Step 1: Gradual Elimination of BPH-Unfriendly Foods

1. **Immediate Action After Diagnosis:**

    Immediately after receiving a BPH diagnosis, take the time to thoroughly assess your existing food inventory at home, ideally within the first week. This initial step is crucial for setting a positive direction for your dietary adjustments.

Work closely with a trusted family member or consult your primary care provider to meticulously identify and eliminate foods known to worsen BPH symptoms, using the detailed list provided in the previous chapter as a guide. This process not only helps in making informed decisions about your diet but also in understanding the direct impact of certain foods on your condition.

2. **Family Involvement and Discussion:**

   It's important to have an open and honest discussion with your family members about the necessary changes in meal preparation and diet that you need to make. Acknowledge that this adjustment might require some sacrifices, such as eliminating processed meats from your diet, and recognize that other members of the household may choose to continue consuming them.

   This step is about finding a balance between your dietary needs and the preferences of others in the family. It highlights the importance of mutual support, understanding, and compromise in managing your condition effectively. Encourage your family to participate in this journey with you, making it a collective effort towards healthier eating habits.

3. **Managing Cravings and Building Willpower:**

   Adapting to a new dietary regimen, especially after being accustomed to a diet rich in red meats, processed foods, and other items that aggravate BPH symptoms, will undoubtedly present challenges. It's natural to experience cravings for these familiar foods. Recognize these cravings as a normal part of the adjustment period.

   However, it's crucial to commit to building your willpower to resist giving in to unhealthy urges. Developing strategies for overcoming these initial cravings is essential for your long-term health. This might involve finding healthier alternatives that satisfy your taste without compromising your condition or setting small, achievable goals that reward your progress.

Successfully overcoming these initial obstacles is a significant achievement and lays the groundwork for making more extensive dietary changes that will support your health and well-being following a BPH diagnosis.

This first step is often the most challenging, as it involves confronting and making changes to established eating habits. However, successfully navigating this stage is foundational for implementing further dietary changes and building a supportive environment that prioritizes your health and well-being.

Step 2: Opt for Healthier Substitutes and Reduce Consumption Where Necessary

Once you've eliminated the primary foods that negatively impact BPH, the next step involves identifying healthier alternatives for the remaining items in your diet. This step recognizes that completely removing certain staples may not be practical or desirable due to family preferences or the essential role some ingredients play in cooking.

1. **Identifying Healthier Alternatives**

   Making smarter choices about what we eat can have a significant impact on our health. Here are some strategies for substituting common items with healthier options:

   Healthy Fats and Oils:

   The type of fat used in cooking plays a crucial role in our overall health. Commonly used cooking oils often contain unhealthy fats that can be detrimental to heart health. A simple switch to healthier options like olive oil can make a big difference.

   Olive oil is renowned for its heart-healthy monounsaturated fats, which can help lower bad cholesterol levels and improve cardiovascular health. For ingredients that are difficult to eliminate, such as dairy products, the goal should be to minimize their consumption.

This can be achieved by selecting dairy products that are lower in saturated fats or by choosing plant-based alternatives that can offer similar textures and flavors without health drawbacks.

Reducing Sodium Intake:

Salt has been a staple in culinary practices for centuries, enhancing the flavor of food in ways that few other seasonings can. However, excessive sodium intake is linked to a host of health issues, including high blood pressure and an increased risk of heart disease.

Completely removing salt from one's diet is neither practical nor desirable, as it would significantly detract from the enjoyment of eating. Instead, focus on reducing sodium consumption by being mindful of the sodium content in pre-packaged and processed foods.

Opt for food products labeled as low sodium, and practice moderation when adding salt during cooking. Additionally, steer clear of notoriously high-sodium foods such as junk food, fast food, and canned goods. By opting for fresh ingredients and controlling the amount of salt used in recipes, it's possible to enjoy delicious meals that are also heart-healthy.

2. Making Conscious Choices

Understanding Practical Limitations:

It's important to recognize and accept that not every food item can, or indeed should, be eliminated from our diets. Essential components like salt and specific oils play pivotal roles in culinary practices, contributing to the overall enjoyment and flavor of meals.

The objective here is not to impose self-punishment or promote extreme dietary restrictions. Instead, the aim is to discover a sustainable balance that prioritizes your health and well-being, while still allowing you to savor the joy and pleasure that comes from eating delicious food.

Adjust Consumption:

When it comes to ingredients that are difficult to substitute, such as dairy products often used in baked goods, the principle of moderation becomes key. It's crucial to be mindful of the quantities we consume and to pay close attention to serving sizes.

In addition, there's an opportunity to experiment with healthier alternatives, like low-fat dairy options, which can be used in baking. This approach not only allows for the enjoyment of baked treats but also supports a healthier lifestyle by reducing the intake of saturated fats without compromising on taste.

The essence of this step is not about complete deprivation but about making smarter dietary choices. By substituting where possible and reducing consumption of less healthy options, you can manage BPH symptoms effectively while still enjoying a diverse and satisfying diet.

Step 3: Enrich Your Diet Through Creativity and Planning

Adjusting your diet after a BPH diagnosis offers an excellent opportunity to invigorate your meals with creativity and variety. This step is essential not only for adhering to dietary restrictions but also for ensuring that your culinary experience remains enjoyable and fulfilling.

1. **Delving into New Recipes**

    Broadening Your Culinary Horizons:

    The thought of following a diet may evoke images of dull, repetitive meals. However, a BPH-friendly diet does not have to be limited or unappealing. On the contrary, it can be an exciting exploration of flavors and cuisines.

Actively seeking out new recipes that fit within BPH dietary guidelines is key to keeping your meals interesting and diverse. This proactive approach will help maintain your enthusiasm and commitment to your dietary changes, making it much simpler to stick with them over time.

Expanding Meal Variety:

Introducing a wide range of dishes can transform your diet from a set of restrictions into a vibrant and satisfying culinary adventure. Experiment with global cuisines that prioritize fresh, whole ingredients and lean proteins, which are not only delicious but also beneficial for managing BPH symptoms. Using herbs, spices, and healthy fats like olive oil can add depth and richness to your dishes without relying on harmful additives or excessive salt.

2. Enhancing Meal Planning

Crafting a Comprehensive Meal Plan:

Begin with crafting a detailed meal plan for the week. This plan should strike a careful balance between meeting dietary requirements and incorporating a selection of exciting, new recipes.

Effective meal planning ensures a controlled intake of potentially problematic foods while encouraging culinary experimentation. It also simplifies grocery shopping, reduces food waste, and assists in managing portion sizes.

Incorporating Themes and Special Nights:

To make meal planning even more engaging, consider introducing themed meal nights or dedicating specific days to exploring particular types of cuisine. This not only makes the planning process enjoyable but also ensures you're getting a balanced diet full of the nutrients necessary to manage your BPH symptoms.

3. Fostering Connections and Pursuing Passions

Engaging Family in Meal Preparation:

Turning meal preparation into a shared endeavor with family members can create meaningful connections and provide substantial emotional support. By involving others in the cooking process, you can share the joys and challenges of adhering to a BPH-friendly diet, making it a more positive experience for everyone involved.

Exploring Culinary Interests:

If cooking is a passion of yours, this dietary shift presents a perfect chance to deepen your culinary knowledge and skills. For those juggling busy schedules, preparing meals in advance is a practical way to ensure you always have healthy, BPH-friendly options on hand, fitting seamlessly into your lifestyle.

Savoring the Journey

It's important to remember that adopting a BPH-friendly diet is not about restriction but rather about discovering new ways to enjoy food while supporting your health. Starting with a simple seven-day meal plan can offer a foundation upon which to build and refine your dietary habits. Look beyond this guide for inspiration, exploring online resources and cookbooks for new recipes that can bring even more variety to your table.

By embedding meal planning and recipe discovery into the core of your approach to managing BPH, you elevate what might initially appear as a daunting adjustment into a valuable opportunity for personal development, familial connection, and, most importantly, enhanced well-being.

Foods to Eat and to Avoid

Managing Benign Prostatic Hyperplasia (BPH) can be significantly influenced by dietary choices. Here's a comprehensive guide on what to eat and what to avoid to support a BPH-friendly diet.

Foods to Eat

When it comes to BPH, maintaining a healthy and balanced diet is crucial. Here are some types of food that can support your overall health and help manage BPH symptoms:

- *Vegetables*: Particularly those high in antioxidants and fiber such as tomatoes (rich in lycopene), bell peppers, broccoli, and leafy greens. These can help reduce inflammation and support overall prostate health.
- *Fruits*: Focus on fruits that are high in vitamins and antioxidants. Berries, like strawberries, raspberries, and blueberries, are excellent choices for their antioxidant properties.
- *Healthy Fats*: Incorporate sources of omega-3 fatty acids, which can be found in flaxseeds, chia seeds,

walnuts, and fatty fish like salmon and mackerel. These fats are beneficial for reducing inflammation.
- *Whole Grains*: Opt for whole grains over refined ones. Foods like oats, brown rice, barley, and quinoa are rich in fiber and nutrients.
- *Legumes*: Beans, lentils, and peas are great plant-based protein sources that are also high in fiber and micronutrients.
- *Protein Sources*: Focus on lean protein sources such as chicken, turkey, and fish. Plant-based proteins like tofu and tempeh are also beneficial.
- *Green Tea*: Contains antioxidants known as catechins, which may help in reducing BPH symptoms.

By incorporating these foods into your diet, you can help support prostate health and potentially improve BPH symptoms.

Foods to Avoid

Following a BPH-friendly diet also means limiting or avoiding certain foods that may worsen symptoms. These include:

- *Sugary Drinks*: Beverages like soda, energy drinks, and sweetened juices are loaded with sugar
- *Red Meat and Processed Meats*: These can increase inflammation and are linked to higher risks of BPH progression.

- ***Dairy Products***: High consumption of dairy products has been associated with an increased risk of developing BPH.
- ***Caffeine and Alcohol***: Both can irritate the bladder and exacerbate BPH symptoms. It's best to limit intake or opt for decaffeinated versions.
- ***Spicy Foods***: While not universally problematic, spicy foods can worsen symptoms for some individuals with BPH.
- ***Sodium-rich Foods***: High sodium intake can contribute to increased BPH symptoms. Avoid processed and pre-packaged foods that tend to be high in sodium.
- ***Sugary Foods and Beverages***: Excessive sugar can lead to weight gain and increase inflammation, adversely affecting BPH conditions.
- ***Trans Fats and Saturated Fats***: Found in fried foods, baked goods, and certain oils, these fats can worsen overall health and BPH symptoms.

A BPH-friendly diet focuses on whole, unprocessed foods rich in antioxidants, fibers, and healthy fats while minimizing the intake of inflammatory foods, caffeine, alcohol, and processed items. Individual responses to certain foods can vary, so it's important to monitor your symptoms and adjust your diet accordingly.

Sample 7-Day Meal Plan

Following a BPH-friendly diet doesn't have to be complicated. Here's a sample 7-day meal plan to help you get started:

Table 1: description

	Morning (breakfast and AM snack)	**Afternoon (lunch and PM snack)**	**Evening**
Day 1	Chia seed and strawberry pudding Fruity berry spinach smoothie	Baked salmon and lentil stew	Ikarian stew with black-eyed peas Sauteed sardines in olive oil
	Strawberries and nuts	Citrus fruits	
Day 2	Salmon with avocados and Brussel sprouts Berry smoothie	Caesar salad and seafood stew	Chicken soup and sauteed asparagus
	Apples and	Walnuts and	

		oranges	almonds	
Day 3		Roasted broccoli and salmon Fruitty berry spinach smoothie	Salmon and asparagus Zucchini and celery greens soup	Broccoli soup Baked salmon
		Chia seed and strawberry pudding	Lemons and grapefruit	
Day 4		Toasted whole wheat bread Salmon soup	Vegetable broth Chicken rotisserie	Salmon with avocado and Brussel sprout Broccoli soup
		Fresh tomato salad	Chia seed and strawberry pudding Fruity berry spinach smoothie	
Day 5		Chicken soup Sauteed asparagus	Ikarian stew with black-eyed peas Baked salmon	Seafood stew Caesar salad
		Peanut butter and whole wheat bread	Walnut and almonds	
Day 6		Broccoli soup Salmon and asparagus	Lentil stew Sauteed sardines in	Chicken rotisserie Vegetable

			olive oil	broth
		Fruitty berry spinach smoothie	Fresh tomato salad	
Day 7		Chia seed and strawberry pudding Salmon soup	Steamed trout and sauteed asparagus	Roasted broccoli and salmon
		Walnuts and almonds	Berries	

The provided meal plan is carefully designed to cater to individuals with BPH, prioritizing foods that offer the most benefits and ease for those with this condition. A heavy emphasis is placed on consuming a variety of fruits and vegetables due to their numerous health advantages for BPH patients.

Each main meal daily combines vegetables with either fish or chicken, deliberately excluding red meats like pork, beef, or lamb to avoid aggravating the condition. While many recommended dishes feature salmon and other types of cold-water fish, those who prefer not to follow a pescatarian diet can choose lean poultry options instead. Poultry serves as an excellent protein source that does not pose the same risks to individuals with BPH as red meat does.

The meal plan emphasizes simplicity in preparation, with ingredients that are generally easy to find. Readers are encouraged to personalize these meals by adding other BPH-friendly ingredients to suit their tastes.

To maintain energy levels and manage appetite throughout the day, snacks are strategically included between main meals. Opting for smaller, more frequent meals is beneficial for those with BPH, as opposed to larger meals eaten less frequently. The recommended snacks, which include nuts and citrus fruits, are specifically chosen for their suitability for BPH patients. For variety, a chicken salad sandwich can serve as a fulfilling snack alternative.

It's important to note that the recipes provided in this meal plan are not exhaustive. Readers are encouraged to explore local dishes or international recipes as a way to diversify their diet further. This approach aligns with the third step of our comprehensive plan, aiming to make the dietary management of BPH both enjoyable and fulfilling.

Tips for Meal Planning and Food Preparation

Following a BPH-friendly diet can be challenging, as it requires careful planning and preparation. To help make this process easier, here are some tips to keep in mind while meal planning and food preparation:

- ***Start with a list***: Before heading to the grocery store, make a list of the ingredients needed for your meals.

This will help you stay organized and focused while shopping.
- *Shop for fresh produce*: Incorporating fruits and vegetables into your diet is crucial for managing BPH symptoms. Make sure to choose fresh produce over canned or processed options whenever possible.
- *Choose lean proteins*: Lean meats like chicken, fish, and tofu are low in saturated fat and beneficial for those with BPH. Other sources of protein include beans, lentils, and eggs.
- *Experiment with spices*: Instead of relying on high-fat or high-sodium sauces and condiments for flavor, try using herbs and spices to add taste to your meals. This is a healthier option and can also provide additional health benefits.
- *Meal prep*: Set aside some time at the beginning of the week to prepare meals in advance. This will save time and effort during busier days, making it easier to stick to your meal plan.
- *Involve others*: Cooking with family or friends can make meal preparation more enjoyable and can also help incorporate new recipes into your meal plan.
- *Don't restrict yourself*: While it's important to follow a healthy and balanced diet, don't restrict yourself too much. Allowing yourself occasional treats or trying new foods can make the dietary management of BPH more sustainable in the long run.

By following these tips, you can create a meal plan that is not only beneficial for managing BPH but also enjoyable and sustainable for your lifestyle. Remember to consult with a healthcare professional or registered dietitian for personalized dietary recommendations for managing BPH.

Sample Recipes

These are just some sample recipes to get you started on your BPH-friendly meal plan. Feel free to make adjustments and add in your favorite ingredients!

Chicken Rotisserie and Vegetable Broth

Ingredients:

- 2 lbs chicken breasts, boneless and skinless
- 1 onion, chopped
- 1 stalk celery, chopped
- 1 carrot, chopped
- 2 cloves garlic, minced
- 4 cups low-sodium chicken broth
- Salt and pepper to taste

Instructions:

1. In a large pot, add the chicken breasts and cover with water. Bring to a boil and let cook for 20 minutes.
2. Remove the chicken from the pot and let cool before shredding it into small pieces.
3. In another pot, sauté the onion, celery, carrot, and garlic until they become tender.
4. Add the shredded chicken back into the pot and continue to sauté for a few more minutes.
5. Pour in the chicken broth and bring to a boil.
6. Reduce heat and let simmer for 30 minutes, adding salt and pepper to taste.
7. Serve hot as a nourishing lunch or light dinner option.

Ikarian Stew with Black-Eyed Peas

Ingredients:

- 2 cups dried black-eyed peas, discard stones and drain and rinse after soaking for an hour
- 2 garlic cloves, minced
- 1 onion, chopped
- 1 fennel bulb, trimmed, halved, and sliced into thin strips
- 4 celery stalks, chopped
- 3 carrots, peeled and chopped
- 1 tomato, diced
- 2 bay leaves
- 3 tbsp. tomato paste
- 1 tsp. salt
- 1/2 cup fresh dill, chopped
- 4 large kale leaves, slivered
- olive oil

Instructions:

1. Drain and rinse the peas before proceeding with the recipe.
2. Place the peas, garlic, onion, carrots, fennel, tomato, and celery in the slow cooker. Cover with water.
3. Add bay leaves, salt, and tomato paste.
4. Place the lid and set it to cook on low for 7 hours.

5. Add the dill and kale leaves about 15-20 minutes before the cooking time is done.
6. Leave to cook until the time is over or until the kale is soft.
7. Season with pepper and salt according to desired taste.
8. Upon serving, drizzle with olive oil and enjoy while hot.

Lentil Stew

Ingredients:

- 4 cups savoy cabbage, chopped
- 1 tbsp. anchovy paste
- 3-1/2 tbsp. extra virgin olive oil
- 2 tsp. cumin
- 1 shallot, chopped finely
- 1 tsp. turmeric
- 1 leek, chopped finely
- 4 carrots, chopped finely
- 2 celery stalks, chopped finely
- pepper
- unrefined sea salt
- 2 cups organic vegetable broth
- 1 26-oz. can of chopped tomatoes, drained
- 2 15-oz. cans of lentils, rinsed and drained
- 1 tbsp. unfiltered and unpasteurized apple cider vinegar
- 1/2 cup parsley, chopped
- 4 organic pasture-raised eggs
- optional: egg topping

Instructions:

1. Boil water in a large pot.
2. Add cabbage and let cook for about 10 minutes, or until soft. Drain after and set aside.

3. In the same pot, pour in oil and place over medium heat.
4. Add the cumin, anchovy paste, shallots, turmeric, celery, carrots, and leeks.
5. Saute for about 8 to 10 minutes, or until the vegetables are soft.
6. Season with salt and pepper, according to your taste.
7. Add the tomatoes and cabbage, and let cook for another 5 minutes.
8. Pour in the vegetable broth and cook for 10 minutes.
9. Add lentils and cook for another 5 minutes.
10. Remove stew from heat, and add parsley.
11. Serve while hot.

Vegetable Broth

Ingredients:

- 1 tbsp. oil
- 2 leeks, sliced
- 2 carrots, sliced
- 2 ribs celery
- 1/4 tsp. salt
- 8 cups water

To make the soup:

- 1 tbsp. oil
- 2 cups potatoes, diced
- 1 cup mushrooms, diced
- 1-1/2 cups cauliflower, diced
- 1 cup onion, diced
- 1 cup celery, diced
- 1 cup carrot, diced
- 1-1/2 cups red beans, cooked
- 2 sprigs of rosemary
- 4 sprigs of thyme
- 2 cups spinach

Instructions:

1. To a pot on medium heat, add oil and leeks.
2. Cook for about three minutes or until they start to soften up.

3. Add carrots and top a few celery stalks with leaves.
4. Cover with water.
5. Add salt. Bring to a simmer and cook until carrots are very tender but not mushy.
6. Turn off the heat and let it cool down a little.
7. When the broth has cooled down, strain out the veggies.
8. Remove carrots and set them aside.
9. Squeeze most of the liquid out of the leeks and celery.

To cook the soup:

1. Add carrots to some of the broth and blend.
2. With a pot on medium heat, add oil, onions, raw carrots, and celery. Cook until onions are translucent, approximately 3 to 5 minutes.
3. Add broth, potatoes, and herbs.
4. Bring to a simmer and cook for 10 minutes.
5. Add cauliflower and red beans.
6. Simmer for another 5 minutes.
7. Add the package of frozen green beans and cook until the potatoes and cauliflower are tender, approximately for another 5 minutes.
8. At the end of cooking, add spinach.
9. Serve warm.

Broccoli Soup

Ingredients:

- 1 onion, chopped
- 1 lb. broccoli, chopped
- 1 small tomato, chopped
- 1 tbsp. grapeseed oil
- 1/2 cup unsweetened almond milk
- 16 oz. water
- 1/4 tsp. turmeric
- cayenne pepper, to taste

Instructions:

1. Put oil and onion in a medium pot. Saute over medium heat for about a couple of minutes.
2. Add the seasoning, tomato, and broccoli. Saute for 10 more minutes.
3. Add 6 ounces of water. Cover the pot and let it simmer for a couple more minutes.
4. Transfer the contents into a blender, followed by the remaining water and milk. Blend for a couple of minutes.
5. Pour back the blended ingredients into the pot.
6. Raise the heat and boil for a couple of minutes.
7. Serve and enjoy while hot.

Chicken Soup

Ingredients:

- 4 cups of low-sodium, fat-free chicken broth
- 2 cups skinless and organic chicken, boiled and diced
- 2 carrots, diced
- 1 red onion, chopped
- 3/4 cup turnip, diced
- 1/2 cup fresh parsley, chopped

Instructions:

1. Using medium heat, boil the chicken broth in a large saucepan.
2. Add the carrots, onion, turnip, and parsley to the broth.
3. Reduce the heat from medium to low. Cover the saucepan.
4. Simmer until the vegetables are tender.
5. Add the diced chicken.
6. Simmer the soup for another 3 to 4 minutes.
7. Serve and enjoy while hot.

Salmon Soup

Ingredients:

- 1-3/4 cup coconut milk
- 2 tsp. dried thyme leaves
- 4 leeks, trimmed and sliced into crescents
- 6 cups seafood stock or chicken broth
- salt, for seasoning
- 3 cloves garlic, minced
- 1 lb. salmon, cut into bite-sized pieces
- 2 tbsp. avocado oil

Instructions:

1. Place avocado oil in a large saucepan or Dutch oven at low-medium heat. Add garlic and leeks.
2. Cook vegetables until slightly softened.
3. Pour in chicken or fish stock. Add in thyme and allow the mixture to simmer for approximately 15 minutes.
4. Season with salt to taste.
5. Add both coconut milk and salmon.
6. Bring the mixture up to a gentle simmer.
7. Cook until the fish is tender and opaque, then serve while hot.

Salmon and Asparagus

Ingredients:

- 2 salmon filets
- 14-oz. young potatoes
- 8 asparagus spears, trimmed and halved
- 2 handfuls cherry tomatoes
- 1 handful of basil leaves
- 2 tbsp. extra-virgin olive oil
- 1 tbsp. balsamic vinegar

Instructions:

1. Heat oven to 428°F.
2. Arrange potatoes into a baking dish.
3. Drizzle potatoes with extra-virgin olive oil.
4. Roast potatoes until they have turned golden brown.
5. Place asparagus into the baking dish together with the potatoes.
6. Roast in the oven for 15 minutes.
7. Arrange cherry tomatoes and salmon among the vegetables.
8. Drizzle with balsamic vinegar and the remaining olive oil.
9. Roast until the salmon is cooked.
10. Throw in basil leaves before transferring everything to a serving dish.
11. Serve while hot.

Seafood Stew

Ingredients:

- 2 tsp. extra-virgin olive oil
- 1 cut bulb fennel
- 2 stalks of celery, chopped
- 2 cups white wine
- 1 tbsp. chopped thyme
- 1 cup chopped shallots
- 6 ounces shrimp
- 6 ounces of sea scallops
- 1/4 tsp. salt
- 1 cup chopped parsley
- 6 oz. Arctic char
- 2-1/2 cups of water

Instructions:

1. Heat a frying pan on the lowest setting. Add a small amount of oil.
2. Cook the celery, shallots, and fennel for approximately 6 minutes.
3. Pour the wine, water, and thyme into the frying pan.
4. Wait for 10 minutes and allow it to cook.
5. Once much of the water has evaporated, add in the remaining ingredients, and wait for 2 minutes before removing it from the stove.
6. Serve and enjoy immediately.

Salmon with Avocados and Brussels Sprouts

Ingredients:

- 2 lbs. of salmon filet, divided into 4 pieces
- 1 tsp. ground cumin
- 1 tsp. onion powder
- 1 tsp. paprika powder
- 1/2 tsp. garlic powder
- 1 tsp. chili powder
- Himalayan sea salt
- black pepper, freshly ground

Avocado sauce:

- 2 chopped avocados
- 1 lime, squeezed for the juice
- 1 tbsp. extra-virgin olive oil
- 1 tbsp. fresh minced cilantro
- 1 diced small red onion
- 1 minced garlic clove
- Himalayan sea salt to taste
- black pepper, freshly ground

Brussels sprouts:

- 3 lbs. of Brussels sprouts
- 1/2 cup raw honey
- 1/2 cup balsamic vinegar
- 1/2 cup melted coconut oil

- 1 cup dried cranberries
- Himalayan sea salt
- black pepper, freshly ground

Instructions:

To make the salmon and avocado sauce:

1. Combine cumin, onion, chili powder, garlic, and paprika seasoned with salt and pepper. Mix well before dry rubbing on the salmon.
2. Place the salmon in the fridge for 30 minutes.
3. Preheat the grill.
4. In a bowl, mash avocado until the texture becomes smooth. Pour in all the remaining ingredients and mix thoroughly.
5. Grill salmon for 5 minutes on each side or until cooked.
6. Drizzle avocado on cooked salmon.

To prepare the Brussels sprouts:

1. Preheat the oven to 375°F.
2. Mix Brussels sprouts with coconut oil. Season with salt and pepper.
3. Place vegetables on a baking sheet and roast for about 30 minutes.

4. In a separate pan, combine vinegar and honey.
5. Simmer in slow heat until it boils and thickens.
6. Drizzle them on top of the Brussels sprouts.
7. Serve with the salmon.

Baked Salmon

Ingredients:

- 2 salmon fillets
- 6 cups of fresh spinach
- 2 tsp. coconut oil
- 1/4 tsp. garlic powder
- 1/4 tsp. turmeric
- 3 large cloves of garlic
- lemon juice
- salt
- pepper

Instructions:

1. Preheat the oven to 400°F.
2. Line a baking dish with parchment paper.
3. Marinate salmon fillets in lemon juice, coconut oil, garlic powder, turmeric, salt, and pepper.
4. Let it sit for a few minutes. This may also be done the night before to help the juices and flavor get into the salmon.
5. Once the oven is ready, bake the salmon for 15 minutes.
6. Cook some of the garlic in a pan with coconut oil.

7. Add spinach and cook until ready. Season with salt and pepper to taste.
8. Take salmon out of the oven and put spinach beside it.
9. Serve and enjoy.

Zucchini and Celery Greens Soup

Ingredients:

- 1/2 cup cooked green lentils
- 1 onion, finely diced
- 1 parsnip, peeled and finely diced
- 2 garlic cloves, crushed
- 1 green bell pepper, cut into small cubes
- 1 zucchini, sliced
- 4 asparagus spears
- 1 fennel bulb, diced finely
- 2 celery stalks, diced finely
- 1 small bunch of celery greens or other greens available: beet greens, kale, or spinach

- 2 cups low-sodium vegetable broth
- 1 lime, juice only
- 1 tsp. Chia seeds to garnish
- freshly ground black pepper

Instructions:

1. In a large saucepan, add the onion, parsnip, garlic, and green bell pepper.
2. Cook on medium heat for 5 minutes until softened. Stir occasionally.
3. Add zucchini and cook for an additional 2 minutes.
4. Pour in the vegetable broth and bring to a boil.

5. Reduce heat to low and simmer for 10 minutes.
6. Add asparagus, fennel, celery stalks, and greens to the soup.
7. Simmer for another 5 minutes until all vegetables are soft.
8. Remove from heat and let cool for a few minutes.
9. Using an immersion blender or regular blender, blend soup until smooth.
10. Add lime juice and black pepper to taste.
11. Serve hot with a sprinkle of chia seeds on top for added texture and nutrition.

Chia Seed and Strawberry Pudding

Ingredients:

- 1 cup strawberries, thinly sliced
- 3 tbsp. chia seeds
- 1 cup soy beverage, unsweetened and fortified

Instructions:

1. To create pudding, combine the soy beverage and chia seeds.
2. Refrigerate the mixture for half an hour. Stir the mixture every 5 minutes to prevent the chia seeds from sticking together.
3. As an alternative, blend the soy beverage and chia seeds in a food processor and let it chill in the refrigerator.
4. Slice strawberries lengthwise.
5. Pour chilled pudding into 2 glasses. Place the strawberry slices on top.
6. Serve and enjoy your pudding.

Fruity Berry Spinach Smoothie

Ingredients:

- 1 cup watermelon
- 1 cup almond milk
- 1/2 small banana
- 1 handful of spinach
- 5 frozen strawberries
- 1 tsp. chia seeds
- 1 cup of ice

Instructions:

1. Mix spinach, banana, chia seeds, half a cup of ice, and a half cup of almond milk. Do this to prevent a brown smoothie.
2. Pour into a glass.
3. Blend the rest of the ingredients.
4. Pour both of the mixtures into the same glass.
5. Serve and enjoy!

Roasted Broccoli and Salmon

Ingredients:

- 1-1/2 lbs. or 1 bunch of broccoli, cut into florets
- 4 tbsp. avocado oil, divided
- 1 tsp salt
- 1 tsp pepper
- 4 pcs. salmon filets, deskinned
- 1 pc. jalapeño or red Fresno chile deseeded and sliced into thin rings
- 2 tbsp. unseasoned rice vinegar
- 2 tbsp. capers drained

Instructions:

1. Preheat the oven to 400° F.
2. Place broccoli florets on a large, rimmed baking sheet. Drizzle with 2 tbsp. avocado oil and season with salt and pepper.
3. Roast the florets in the oven for 12 or 15 minutes. Toss occasionally.
4. Remove from the oven when the florets are crisp-tender and browned.
5. Gently rub the salmon filets with 1 tbsp. of the avocado oil. Season with salt and pepper.
6. Place the salmon in the middle of the baking sheet. Move the florets to the sides of the baking sheet.

7. Roast the filet for 10 to 15 minutes or until the filets turn opaque throughout.
8. In a small bowl, combine the vinegar, chile rings, and a pinch of salt. Let the mixture sit for about 10 minutes, allowing the chile rings to soften a bit.
9. Add the capers and the remaining avocado oil. Add salt and pepper to taste.
10. Drizzle chile vinaigrette over the roasted broccoli and salmon just before serving.

Tomato and Spinach Quinoa Salad

Ingredients:

- 1 cup quinoa
- 2 cups water or low-sodium vegetable broth
- 1 cup cherry tomatoes, halved
- 2 cups fresh spinach, chopped
- 1/4 cup red onion, finely chopped
- 1/4 cup cucumber, diced
- 1/4 cup olive oil
- 2 tablespoons lemon juice
- Salt (optional) and pepper to taste
- Fresh basil leaves for garnish

Instructions:

1. Rinse quinoa under cold running water until the water runs clear.
2. In a medium saucepan, bring water or broth to a boil. Add quinoa, reduce heat to low, cover, and simmer for 15 minutes or until all liquid is absorbed.
3. Remove from heat and fluff with a fork. Allow to cool slightly.
4. In a large bowl, combine cooled quinoa, cherry tomatoes, spinach, red onion, and cucumber.

5. In a small bowl, whisk together olive oil, lemon juice, salt (if using), and pepper. Pour over the salad and toss to coat evenly.
6. Garnish with fresh basil leaves before serving.

Lemon-Garlic Baked Salmon

Ingredients:

- 4 salmon fillets
- 2 tablespoons olive oil
- 2 cloves garlic, minced
- 2 tablespoons lemon juice
- Zest of 1 lemon
- 1 teaspoon dried dill or fresh dill to taste
- Salt (optional) and pepper to taste
- Lemon slices for serving

Instructions:

1. Preheat oven to 375°F.
2. In a small bowl, whisk together olive oil, minced garlic, lemon juice, lemon zest, dried dill (or fresh dill), and salt (if using).
3. Place salmon fillets in a baking dish or on a lined baking sheet.
4. Pour the marinade over the salmon and use a spoon to spread it evenly over the fillets.
5. Bake for 15-20 minutes, or until salmon is cooked through and flakes easily with a fork.
6. Serve with lemon slices on top for extra flavor and presentation.

Chicken and Broccoli Stir-Fry

Ingredients:

- 1 tablespoon olive oil
- 2 chicken breasts, sliced into strips
- 2 cups broccoli florets
- 1 red bell pepper, sliced
- 2 cloves garlic, minced
- 1 tablespoon low-sodium soy sauce or tamari
- 1 tablespoon water
- 1 teaspoon sesame oil
- Salt (optional) and pepper to taste
- Sesame seeds for garnish

Instructions:

1. In a large skillet or wok, heat olive oil over medium-high heat.
2. Add chicken strips and cook until browned on all sides, about 5-7 minutes.
3. Add broccoli florets, red bell pepper slices, and minced garlic to the skillet. Cook for an additional 5 minutes.
4. In a small bowl, mix soy sauce, water, and sesame oil. Pour the mixture over the chicken and vegetables in the skillet.

5. Stir-fry for an additional 3-4 minutes until the chicken is fully cooked and the vegetables are tender.
6. Season with salt (if using) and pepper to taste.
7. Serve hot, garnished with sesame seeds if desired.

Avocado and Bean Wrap

Ingredients:

- 2 whole grain wraps
- 1 ripe avocado, mashed
- 1 cup canned low-sodium black beans, rinsed and drained
- 1/2 cup corn kernels (fresh or frozen and thawed)
- 1/4 cup red onion, finely chopped
- 1/4 cup tomato, diced
- Juice of 1 lime
- Salt (optional) and pepper to taste
- Fresh cilantro leaves for garnish

Instructions:

1. Lay out the two whole-grain wraps on a clean surface.
2. In a small bowl, mix mashed avocado, black beans, corn kernels, red onion, tomato, and lime juice.
3. Divide the mixture evenly between the two wraps and spread it over one-half of each wrap.
4. Season with salt (if using) and pepper to taste.
5. Roll the wrap tightly, tucking in the sides as you go.
6. Heat a non-stick skillet over medium heat and lightly spray with cooking oil.

7. Place the wraps seam side down in the skillet and cook for 2-3 minutes on each side until lightly browned and crispy.
8. Serve warm, garnished with fresh cilantro leaves.

Conclusion

Congratulations and heartfelt thanks for dedicating your time to complete this insightful guide on managing Benign Prostatic Hyperplasia (BPH) through diet. Your commitment to exploring and understanding the nutritional avenues for alleviating BPH symptoms showcases a proactive approach toward your health, something truly commendable.

Navigating through the complex relationship between diet and BPH, this guide has armed you with the knowledge to make informed dietary choices that support prostate health. The insights you've gathered are more than just guidelines; they are stepping stones towards a lifestyle that harmonizes with your body's needs, fostering well-being and symptom management.

One of the most pivotal insights from our exploration is the undeniable impact of whole, nutrient-dense foods on your health. Integrating a variety of fruits, vegetables, whole grains, and lean proteins into your daily routine can significantly influence your body's ability to manage inflammation and hormonal balances, both of which are crucial in managing BPH symptoms. This approach isn't just about avoiding discomfort; it's about enhancing your overall vitality and longevity.

We also uncovered the importance of hydration and the mindful consumption of beverages. Water is your best ally, facilitating urinary functions and potentially easing the discomfort associated with BPH. On the flip side, caffeine and alcohol can exacerbate symptoms, making moderation or avoidance a wise choice for many.

Another critical takeaway is the synergy between diet and lifestyle. Regular physical activity complements your dietary efforts, amplifying the benefits to your prostate health and beyond. It's a holistic approach where each positive habit builds upon the other, creating a foundation for healthier living.

Implementing these dietary changes requires patience, resilience, and adaptability. It's a process of discovery, learning how your body responds to different foods and adjusting accordingly. Celebrate every small victory along this journey, for each step forward is a triumph over BPH.

It's also vital to remember that everyone's body is unique. What works for one person may not work for another. Listen to your body, noting how it reacts to certain foods and adjusting your diet to suit your individual needs. This personalized approach ensures that you're doing what's best for your body and your symptoms.

You are not alone on this path. Countless others are navigating the same challenges, seeking ways to manage BPH through diet and lifestyle adjustments. There's a community of support out there—doctors, nutritionists, and fellow BPH sufferers—all united in the goal of finding relief and improving quality of life. Don't hesitate to reach out, share your experiences, and learn from others.

By now, you understand that managing BPH through diet isn't just about mitigating symptoms—it's about adopting a healthier lifestyle that benefits every aspect of your well-being. It's a commitment to nourishing your body, respecting its needs, and treating it with care.

Keep pushing forward with the insights and strategies you've learned. Experiment, adjust, and find what works best for you. And most importantly, stay positive. The path to managing BPH through diet is a marathon, not a sprint. It requires persistence, but every positive change, no matter how small, is a step in the right direction.

Thank you once again for taking the time to explore the potential of diet in managing BPH. Your effort to educate yourself and take action is a powerful testament to your commitment to health. Keep moving forward, fueled by the knowledge that you're doing everything in your power to support your prostate health and overall well-being.

Remember, the road to improvement is paved with challenges, but it's also filled with opportunities for growth and healing. You have the tools and understanding to make a significant impact on your health. Stay motivated, stay informed, and above all, stay hopeful. Here's to your health, happiness, and a brighter, symptom-free future.

FAQ

What foods should i eat to help manage BPH symptoms?

Focus on a diet rich in fruits, vegetables, whole grains, and lean proteins. Specific foods that might be beneficial include tomatoes (rich in lycopene), berries (packed with antioxidants), and fish high in omega-3 fatty acids like salmon and mackerel. These foods can help reduce inflammation and support overall prostate health.

Are there foods i should avoid to prevent worsening BPH symptoms?

Yes, certain foods and beverages can exacerbate BPH symptoms. Try to limit or avoid caffeine, alcohol, spicy foods, and high-sodium foods, as these can increase urinary frequency and discomfort. Reducing the intake of red meat and dairy products might also be beneficial for some individuals.

How much water should i drink daily?

Hydration is crucial, but balancing it to avoid aggravating BPH symptoms is key. Aim for 6 to 8 glasses of water daily, but try not to consume large amounts of fluid at once or drink too much before bedtime to minimize nighttime urination.

Can dietary changes alone manage BPH symptoms?

While dietary changes can significantly impact BPH symptom management, they are most effective when combined with other treatments or lifestyle adjustments recommended by your healthcare provider. Always consult with a healthcare professional for a comprehensive approach to managing BPH.

Do supplements help in managing BPH symptoms?

Certain supplements, such as saw palmetto, beta-sitosterol, and pygeum, have been studied for their potential benefits in managing BPH symptoms. However, results are mixed, and it's essential to consult with a healthcare provider before starting any supplements to ensure they are appropriate for your situation and won't interfere with other medications.

How quickly will i notice improvement in my symptoms after changing my diet?

The effect of dietary changes on BPH symptoms varies among individuals. Some may notice improvements within a few weeks, while for others, it might take longer. Consistency is key, and maintaining dietary changes as part of an overall healthy lifestyle is critical for long-term management.

Is it necessary to completely eliminate certain foods from my diet?

Not necessarily. Moderation is important. While certain foods may trigger symptoms, eliminating them might not be necessary. Pay attention to how your body responds to different foods and adjust your diet accordingly. Balancing your diet while still enjoying a variety of foods is possible with mindful eating and portion control.

References and Helpful Links

Ng, M., Leslie, S. W., & Baradhi, K. M. (2024, January 11). Benign prostatic hyperplasia. StatPearls - NCBI Bookshelf. https://www.ncbi.nlm.nih.gov/books/NBK558920/

Enlarged prostate: Does diet play a role? (2022, July 2). Mayo Clinic. https://www.mayoclinic.org/diseases-conditions/benign-prostatic-hyperplasia/expert-answers/enlarged-prostate-and-diet/faq-20322773

Tessa. (2021, August 4). Diet and Lifestyle's Impact on your BPH Symptoms | Austin Urology Institute. Austin Urology Institute. https://austinurologyinstitute.com/blog/diet-and-lifestyles-impact-on-your-bph-symptoms/

Espinosa, G. (2013). Nutrition and benign prostatic hyperplasia. Current Opinion in Urology, 23(1), 38–41. https://doi.org/10.1097/mou.0b013e32835abd05

Marcin, A. (2023, March 24). 4 types of foods to avoid for prostate health. Healthline. https://www.healthline.com/health/prostate-cancer/foods-to-avoid-for-prostate-health

Kim, T., Lim, H., Kim, M., & Lee, M. S. (2012). Dietary supplements for benign prostatic hyperplasia: An overview of systematic reviews. Maturitas, 73(3), 180–185. https://doi.org/10.1016/j.maturitas.2012.07.007

Λάγιου, Π., Wuu, J., Trichopoulou, A., Hsieh, C. C., Adami, H., & Trichopoulos, D. (1999). Diet and benign prostatic hyperplasia: a study in Greece. Urology, 54(2), 284–290. https://doi.org/10.1016/s0090-4295(99)00096-5

Harvard Health. (2020, January 29). 10 diet & exercise tips for prostate health. https://www.health.harvard.edu/mens-health/10-diet-and-exercise-tips-for-prostate-health

www.ingramcontent.com/pod-product-compliance
Lightning Source LLC
LaVergne TN
LVHW010410070526
838199LV00065B/5938